MW01014913

BABY SLEEP TRAINING IN 3 DAYS

THE STEP-BY-STEP PLAN TO TEACH YOUR BABY TO CRYING AND SLEEP ALL NIGHT

© **Copyright 2016 by Jenny Simpson - All rights reserved.**

This document is geared towards providing exact and reliable information in regards to the topic and issue covered. The publication is sold with the idea that the publisher is not required to render accounting, officially permitted, or otherwise, qualified services. If advice is necessary, legal or professional, a practiced individual in the profession should be ordered.

- From a Declaration of Principles which was accepted and approved equally by a Committee of the American Bar Association and a Committee of Publishers and Associations.

In no way is it legal to reproduce, duplicate, or transmit any part of this document in either electronic means or in printed format. Recording of this publication is strictly prohibited and any storage of this document is not allowed unless with written permission from the publisher. All rights reserved.

The information provided herein is stated to be truthful and consistent, in that any liability, in terms of inattention or otherwise, by any usage or abuse of any policies, processes, or directions contained within is the solitary and utter responsibility of the recipient reader. Under no circumstances will any legal responsibility or blame be held against the publisher for any reparation, damages, or monetary loss due to the information herein, either directly or indirectly.

Respective authors own all copyrights not held by the publisher.

The information herein is offered for informational purposes solely, and is universal as so. The presentation of the information is without contract or any type of guarantee assurance.

The trademarks that are used are without any consent, and the publication of the trademark is without permission or backing by the trademark owner. All trademarks and brands within this book are for clarifying purposes only and are the owned by the owners themselves, not affiliated with this document.

CONTENTS

SECTION 1

CHAPTER 1 – INTRODUCTION

Being a parent is one of the most amazing feelings you will experience... but these feelings can come crashing down in a heap when your baby won't sleep consistently or on their own, or **at all!** (or so it feels)

Lack of sleep for both baby and parent can be detrimental to relationships and mental health. And if you don't address the issue of sleep when your little one is a baby then it **will** continue through to the toddler stage and beyond.

The great news is that whatever stage your baby is at, my proven **Five Minute Sleep Method** will work and will give you and your little one the tools for healthy sleep habits going forward – to fall asleep quickly, on their own and sleep through the night.

Is my baby 'Normal'?
Let me start by saying there is no such thing as 'normal' when it comes to babies.

They are all so different and unique, yet still we are constantly comparing them, and hoping that ours are 'normal' or even more advanced or special than the other.

Hearing stories of babies who have slept through the night from just a few weeks old and who have no trouble falling asleep can get you down and feeling like you are doing something wrong.

Believe me – these stories are often exaggerated, or if they are in fact true then these same babies will no doubt have issues with sleep later down the track once they have hit a different developmental milestone.

It is true that some babies are 'better' at sleeping than others. You may have been asked if your baby is a 'good baby' or a 'good sleeper'.

From my research, only around 20% of babies are 'easy' in this respect, and these few babies learn how to fall asleep fairly easily.

But, this means there is a huge 80% of babies who need more help to learn the crucial life skill of falling asleep and resettling.

I often tell new parents that they will experience difficulties with their children at one stage or another – whether it be a baby who won't sleep, an unruly toddler or a rebellious teenager, it will happen at some stage. Think on the brightside, and think of yourself as lucky for having a baby who won't sleep - **this is temporary** and you are getting this difficult stage over and done with at such a young age, the rest will seem like smooth sailing from here on in.

Lack of sleep for a parent can exasperate the thoughts of doubt and worry about whether you are doing a good enough job as a parent. It is especially true for first time parents, who often have not had a great deal of experience with babies.

You go through the 40 weeks of pregnancy thinking you are getting all prepared for a new baby to enter your lives, and you picture what life will soon be like.

You never imagined it would be this hard or that your baby would cause so many thoughts of doubt.

You wonder at times if you have even done the right thing by becoming a parent – these thoughts are completely understandable and the majority of parents will experience thoughts like this at one point or another.

You are in a great position having purchased this product to learn the tools to sort any sleep issue at any age or stage for your baby.

> *Don't compare your baby or toddler to any other child, each is unique with very different needs and abilities.*

It's not your fault.

An unsettled or difficult baby doesn't come from a result of the actions of the mother during pregnancy, labour or birth.

Whether the mother ate a lot of chocolate or broccoli during pregnancy or whether a baby is born vaginally or by caesarean section will not affect the likelihood of having a difficult or unsettled baby

Sarah had a wonderful pregnancy, she had no issues with falling pregnant, all of her scans and tests during pregnancy were perfect. She practiced yoga weekly and ate the recommended healthy pregnancy diet. Sarah's labour was a few hours long, no pain relief was required and Baby Sophia was born naturally with no complications. The first 10 days were great; she fed well, slept well and seemed to be a happy baby. Then the bubble burst and life suddenly became very difficult for both Sarah and Sophia. Sophia wouldn't sleep or even stop crying unless she was on Sarah in a baby carrier or feeding on the breast.

Michaela had difficulty falling pregnant having suffered a tragic miscarriage along the journey. When she eventually did fall pregnancy one of the scans showed some abnormalities as well as a possible heart development issue. Michaela was under carefeul obstetric and gynaecological care through the pregnancy. She gained weight and was stressed out and worried about the health of her unborn baby. When Baby Billie was getting ready to enter the world his heart rate dropped and the doctors decided an emergency caesarean section birth was the best option. Billie was born and was taken straight to the neonatal unit at the hospital while Michaela was surgically repaired from the caesarean section. When mum and baby were finally reunited Billie fed perfectly and slept like an angel, and this has continued ever since.

There are of course things you can do assist with the health of your baby during pregnancy and labour, as well as in the early minutes, hours, days and even months of your baby's life.

But things don't always go to plan and ultimately it comes down to the baby's **personality** and development as to how your baby will react to life on the outside.

Whether you feel ripped off because you did everything by the book, or even if you feel as though you have done something wrong by your baby to be in this predicament, there is a solution to every problem you are facing and all bad habits can be reversed.

By searching out and purchasing this program shows you are an attentive, caring parent who wants the best for your baby. You are doing the best thing possible for your baby by giving your baby the gift of sleep.

The word **'new'** in the word **'new**born' is very important. These little creatures are brand *new* to the world and need a lot of comfort and guidance.

> *I remember very clearly being in the hospital when my first child was born. The midwives and nurses took my baby to settle him and give me a break so I could sleep for an hour or two uninterrupted. They returned 20 minutes later telling me that they couldn't settle him and all he needed was his mum – me...... I was completely new to this, I thought, 'If these experts can't get him to settle to sleep then how on earth am I meant to do it?!' It turned out he really did need me, to use my motherly instincts and to simply hear my voice of reassurance.*

Teaching your baby to fall asleep independently and sleep soundly through the night is one of the greatest gifts you can give your precious baby. Sleep is so incredibly important that we spend around one third of our entire life asleep, so let's teach your little one how to fall asleep efficiently and peacefully.

You will feel so much better for it and you will have a happy rested baby.

Learning how to fall asleep and stay asleep all night is a crucial life skill for your baby.

Without a good night's sleep and appropriate naps through the day your baby can't possibly take in and learn from the big wide world rapidly opening up around them - so let's get this bump in the parenting road smoothed out quickly!

I know from my own experience as a mom as well as interviewing and speaking with other mothers, that although each family is different and unique, we all want the same for our children, for them to be healthy and happy. This common goal all starts with the basis of a good night's sleep.

If we can help our children learn this skill then the rest will naturally follow. There will always be bumps along the road in parenthood but we can face it all in a much more relaxed and calm manner if we are all well rested.

Parents often joke when they are handed their beautiful new bundle of joy 'where is the manual for bringing up this baby?' Well there certainly isn't a big book that will fix any parenting issue that will ever arise, but this guide to teaching your baby how to get a good night's sleep is as good as a 'baby manual'.

Once you have sleep sorted, the rest will follow naturally. You will also have much more confidence that you are a great parent and are the decision maker in your baby's life at the moment.

> *Take a t-shirt or singlet that you have been wearing and place it in the bassinette or crib for your baby to sleep on top of. This will smell like you and your baby will feel that you are close and be comforted.*

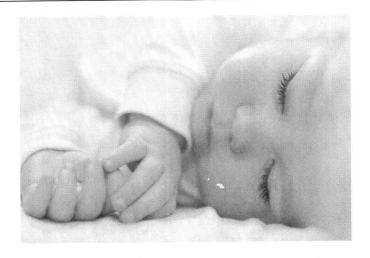

CHAPTER 2 – YOU ARE THE TEACHER

It is really important to let your baby know that you are the teacher and decision maker, you need to take control of the situation.

Yes – we need to follow baby's cues such as tired signals (rubbing eyes, yawning, jerking movements in younger babies, losing focus etc) however these little ones are very new to this sleep business and need our guidance and expertise.

Babies thrive when they feel safe and secure, so trust your instincts and have faith that what you are doing is the right thing for your little one.

> *Believe in your abilities as a parent, your baby will certainly pick up on your confidence and will feel safe and secure in your guidance.*

Many people don't realise that the majority of babies need to *learn* how to fall asleep. For a task that seems as though it should come naturally to all humans, surprisingly the actual process of falling asleep takes some **time** and **teaching**.

Falling asleep is one thing, but falling asleep **quickly** and **on your own**is another.

Sleep is a fairly complicated thing once you look in to the science of it......

All humans wake multiple times during the night as we fall in and out of sleep cycles. We all do it every night, however we have *learnt* how to fall back to sleep and for the majority of the time we don't even remember waking at all during the night.

Do you ever notice that when you wake in the morning that you have taken your socks off, or removed a blanket during the night 'in your sleep'?

Well, you're actually awake and in between sleep cycles. You have learnt over time to quickly fall back to sleep in to the next sleep cycle and generally don't remember waking at all.

Babies who rely on their parents to fall asleep at the start of a nap or the night sleep will then require their parent to be right there to help lull them back to sleep when they also wake in between sleep cycles. This is the key reason to **teach** your baby to fall asleep without you.

Lorraine thought she was doing a great job with Baby Jethro's sleep during the first weeks of his life. He would fall asleep on her breast, and she would transfer him to his crib ever so carefully. He would wake a few times during the night at which time Lorraine would jump up, change and feed him, where he would once again fall straight back asleep on the breast to be transferred asleep to the crib once again. This process continued to the morning.

A few months in to Jethro's life, Lorraine was irritable from lack of solid blocks of sleep, and Jethro was completely reliant on his mum to fall asleep. He was waking up through the night out of habit and was being fed back to sleep, not because he needed the milk feed, but because he needed the comfort of the breast to fall back in to the next sleep cycle. Something needed to change as both mum and baby were not happy or well rested.

During this sleep teaching process you may feel guilty at times and feel like they think you have abandoned them - these feelings are completely normal.

I can assure you that their love and affection for you will only grow and in fact they will be happier and much more content after their full night's sleep. In fact, babies thrive on their parents' leadership and confidence so your relationship will improve.

And remember – the Five Minute Sleep Method has options for not leaving your baby alone in the room.

There have been many studies completed on sleep training, and while much of the evidence contradicts each other, there are no reports that I have come across that show that teaching your baby to fall asleep on their own has any negative effect on the relationship between the baby and parents.

If your baby is used to being fed or rocked to sleep, or having another form of 'sleep prop', they may well be a bit confused on the first or second night of the Five Minute Sleep Method.

A bit of resistance is to be expected.....but babies are very fast learners and will adjust quickly. Just think about how quickly they are learning and adjusting to all other aspects of life, and they cope with so much change.

Other people around you may have strong opinions one way or the other when it comes to teaching your baby the skill of sleep. Remember again that you are your baby's teacher and decision maker, and you know what is best for you and your family.

Trust your instincts and remember that you don't have to justify your decisions to anyone – although you may find it hard to keep quiet about your success once you and your little one are fully rested!

Keep in mind also that you are teaching a crucial life skill, your baby won't understand the importance of this life lesson at this stage of their life, but they will certainly be reaping the rewards very quickly.

> *'There was never a child so lovely, but his mother was glad to get him to sleep.' Ralph Waldo Emerson*

Teaching your baby to fall asleep on their own is the only way to get them to sleep through the night.

Some babies learn quickly in only a couple of nights other may take 5-7 nights.

It is extremely vital that all caregivers of the child are on the same page when it comes to teaching your baby how to sleep.

> *Discuss this and other parenting decisions with your partner and agree on a solution to **together.***

When learning the Five Minute Sleep Method; you, as the teacher and decision maker, will choose whether you stay in the room with your little one or leave them for brief periods.

Whichever option you choose, you need to be in agreement with the other parent and support each other. The first one or two nights may be difficult so working as a team is really important.

Be confident in your decisions and this sleep method and it will pay off.

This process will take commitment and at times may not be easy. Once you have decided on a sleep method, it is important to stick to your plan with a united front. Always keeping in mind that this will guide your baby and ultimately give them the greatest gift of all – the gift of a good night's sleep!

> *Try to get outside at least once a day, fresh air and sunshine helps with your sanity, and also helps your baby's body*

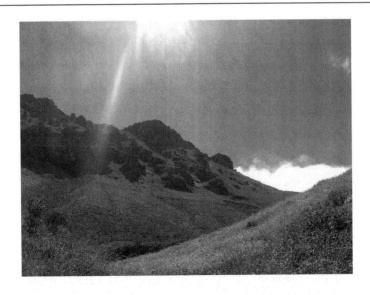

CHAPTER 3 – CHANGES THROUGH THE MONTHS

Once you feel like you've got this baby sleep business down, your little one will change!

> *'Having a baby is one of the most wonderful things in your life, as well as the hardest thing in your life.' Nuno Bettencourt*

You may need to give your baby a refresher course of the Five Minute Sleep Method every so often, this is normal.

It is really easy to slip back in to old habits.

For example when your baby has a cold they can find it difficult to sleep well due to breathing difficulties and generally feeling unwell. During times like these it can be important to be attentive during the night and go to your baby when they cry out for your help. Often what happens though is after only a short period of a couple of nights of this happening your baby will pick up on the fact that your will come running to check on them when they wake and will begin to continue this even when they are well again.

Christina had completed the Five Minute Sleep Method with her 7 month old Jessie and was enjoying hassle free bedtimes and 11 hour stretches of sleep through the night. All her problems had been fixed – at least she thought. For 10 weeks she enjoyed the bliss of evenings to herself and was beginning to feel like life was getting back to 'normal'.

Then Jessie picked up a cold, along with that came as ear infection and burst ear drum. Jessie was waking up in the night with a sore ear after the pain relief medication had worn off. Of course Christina was going to Jessie to comfort her through the night, and resettle. After 3 nights Jessie was feeling much better and back to her bubbly self during the day. But nighttimes were an issue and Christina felt like she was back at square one as Jessie was calling out in the night expecting Christina to come to resettle her has she had done the previous week when she wasn't feeling well.

Just two nights of the refresher course of the Five Minute Sleep Method and both Christina and Jessie were right back on track, as easy as that!

It is often surprising how quickly these bad habits form, but the great news is that as quickly as they form they can be broken. These challenges can be referred to as 'sleep regressions'. After a night or two back using the Five Minute Sleep Method you and your little one will be back on track.

Not only is this true during times of illness but also during other developmental milestones.

Your baby is developing so quickly both physically and mentally.

Let's first look at physical developments and changes.

When babies learn a new skill such as rolling over, sitting up or standing up this too can affect sleep and at times may require a refresher on learning the skill of sleep to get back to the all important goal of sleeping through the night.

A newly learned physical skill can take time to master and come to terms with for your baby.

A baby may have learnt to pull themselves up to a standing position. Their world is now a very different place. Their perceptions have completely changed and their world has suddenly opened up immensely.

It is only natural that this huge change will also affect their sleep.

Once a baby learns how to pull themselves up on the crib to a standing position they may find it difficult to lie back down and get to sleep. Sitting down and lying back down are skills that are generally learnt after sitting and pulling up, you can help the process by giving your little one lots of help and practice during the day with sitting back down safely.

As with any physical change to your baby, you can expect a 'regression' in their sleep.

This can be a shock to the system once you and baby have become used to a full night's sleep. Simply run through the Five Minute Sleep Method refresher course and you will be back on track in no time.

As mentioned, not only is your baby reaching physical developmental milestones, they are also rapidly developing and changing mentally.

Very quickly their world can change.

At birth a baby's brain is about a quarter of the weight of an adult brain. During the first few years of life the brain changes and develops by creating hundreds of billions of cells and cellular connections. So it's no wonder they have periods of being unsettled, there is a lot going on in their brain.

To start with, babies just need to adjust to life on the outside, this in itself is a big change, realising that they are their own being and are in (somewhat) control of their bodies.

Next they learn that they can change and affect the world around them by using their bodies and newly found voices. And from here their brain is developing so significantly and rapidly that what they thought was a safe and secure world one day could suddenly be turned upside down. The only constant in their world is their parents or others close to them.

It is no wonder then that during these periods of change and mental growth that their sleep is affected.

Remember also that all babies develop and change at different paces. In regards to physical developments, some babies may be walking at 9 months, others are closer to 18 months. And the same goes for mental developments; some may be saying words at 8 months, others around 12 months, or later for multi-lingual babies. As long as your baby is developing and learning then try not to compare your baby with other little ones.

Babies and toddlers often suffer pain and discomfort with teething and growing pains. They may be fine during the days when they are up and about but teething pain can often be worse at sleep times as when it comes to sleep time.

Why is this? Well it can often be to do with more blood flow to the area when they are lying down.

Growing pains are another issue that seems to flair up at night time. During the day little ones are moving and distracted, then it comes time to sleep and they slow down and are suddenly aware of the pain.

Analgesics such as children's ibuprofen (Nurofen) and paracetamol (Pamol) are great to use when things are really bad and your little one is in a lot of pain. Just remember to follow the instructions and not to use constantly.

As with any health and wellbeing concerns, if you are worried about the development of your child it is important to seek the opinion of a medical professional.

CHAPTER 4 – HOW MUCH SLEEP DOES MY BABY ACTUALLY NEED?

> *'The nicest thing for me is sleep, then at least I can dream.'* Marilyn Monroe

It is a great idea to create a sleep log to see how your baby is currently sleeping. There is likely more of a pattern than you think.

To do this you can either download a simple application on to your smart phone, there are a few good ones out there where you just click 'Asleep' and then 'Awake' and the app will plot the sleep pattern out on a grid for you. Search for 'Baby Sleep Patterns'.

Alternatively it is really simple just to jot down the times yourself on a piece of paper, or use my simple template below by shading in the times that you baby is asleep:

	6am	8am	10a	12p	2pm	4pm	6pm	8pm	10p	12a	2am	4am
Mon												
Tues												
Wed												
Thurs												
Fri												
Sat												
Sun												

Over a week a so you will probably notice that there is more of a pattern than you realise.

It is important to remember that many babies won't sleep at a particular time each day, rather that they are awake for a certain amount of time before they need to go back to sleep. In the next chapter I will go in to this in more detail.

Sleep times need to be flexible.

Look for the amount of time your baby is awake during the day before they are asleep for their next nap. If for example there is around 2 hours between naps then you can prepare in advance for the next nap, if it is going to be in the pram, car or home.

At night times too, take note of the waking, it could be that the temperature drops at a certain time in your baby's bedroom. An easy solution is to have a heater on a timer to come on prior to the temperature drop to keep baby comfortable. In 'Section 2, Chapter 6' you will also learn how to combat early morning waking.

The below is a **guideline only** for how much a baby might be sleeping, some will require more, others won't need nearly as much.

If your baby is currently sleeping much more or much less than this, remember to not worry – if your baby is healthy and developing well then that is all that matters, don't get hung up on comparing to another baby of a similar age.

We are looking at total hour's sleep, so your baby may be getting a good number of hours sleep, but it may be broken sleep. This is where the frustration occurs and why you are feeling so tired. Don't panic, we will sort that out in 'Section 1 Chapter 6', The Sleep Training

A **0 to 6 week** old baby requires approximately 18 hours sleep a day.
This may consist of
8-10 hours total at night 8-10 hours total at naps
and may include 3-5 naps per day.

A **6 weeks to 6 months** old baby requires approximately 15 hours sleep a day. This may consist of
10 hours total at night
4-5 hours total at naps
and may include 3-4 naps per day.

A **6 months to 12 month** old baby requires approximately 14 hours sleep a day. This may consist of
10-12 hours total at night
2-3 hours total at naps
and may include 2 naps per day.

A **12 month to 18 month** old toddler requires approximately 13 hours sleep a day. This may consist of
11-12 hours at night
2 hours at naps 1 nap per day

An **18 months to 2 year** old toddler requires approximately 13 hours sleep a day. This may consist of
11 hours at night
2 hours at naps
and may include 1 nap per day

A **2 – 3 year** old toddler requires approximately 13 hours sleep a day. This may consist of
11 hours at night
1-2 hours at naps
and may include 1 nap per day.

Please remember once again this is a guideline. Some toddlers have dropped their naps altogether before they turn 2, others may still need 2 naps at 18 months old.

Claire was so worried about the amount of sleep that 10 month old Alexia was getting she thought she couldn't possibly be resting enough for her brain to 'recharge' and take in all of the information she was supposed to be. She created a sleep log and found that the total hours of night sleep was averaging around nine and a half hours, and during the day she was having 2 naps, one in the morning of 1 hour 45 minutes, and one in the afternoon of 40 minutes.

The total amount of sleep was enough for Alexia but Claire was exhausted from the many night wakings and felt she was spending so much of her day and night coaxing Alexia to sleep. Her back was constantly aching from leaning over Alexia's crib to rub her back to help her fall asleep. After 6 nights of using The Baby Sleep Training, and without leaving Alexia alone to cry at all, both mum and baby were enjoying the benefits. Alexia was able to be placed in her crib at the correct time to fall asleep quickly and on her own. During the day Claire was able to enjoy her extra time rather than spending over an hour across the two naps helping Claire fall asleep, and evenings were back to enjoying time with her husband.

CHAPTER 5 – SLEEP TIMINGS

I don't offer 'Sleep Schedule Examples' where there is a list of times that a baby or toddler should be sleeping every day at a particular age. The reason I don't is because this is simply an unachievable task!

Not all babies of one year old will wake at the same time, go for naps at the same time and go to bed at the same time. It's ridiculous to try to fit all babies in to this mould.

Rather than trying to stick to a rigid time schedule, I like to focus more on the *time between* sleeps.

> *During the hour before bed time, turn the lights down and turn off the television and devices. Play some soothing calming music such as Brahms Lullaby.*

This is where **The Gap Effect** comes in.

A baby can generally stay awake for a certain time period before they need to go back to bed again.

The key is finding this awake time period for each particular baby. Some babies and toddlers show very definite signs that they are ready to go to bed, others are a little tougher to pick.

Younger babies generally have a different cry when they are tired. A hungry cry (or just the need to suck) often sounds like a 'naa'or 'neh' – this is because their tongues are making a shape to simulate sucking. A tired cry sounds more like 'aow' – their mouths are simulating more of a yawn and can start with more of a grizzle.

Old babies may rub their eyes or stare blankly in to space as if to 'zone out'.

Toddlers get cranky (although they can be cranky when they're not tired also!).

Others show no obvious signs at all.

Use my grid template in Section 1, Chapter 4 to see if there is a consistent time gap between sleeps.

Once you have this time gap between naps figured out you will notice that as the months go on this gap will increase slightly.

The gap between the last nap of the day and bedtime can sometimes be slightly longer than the gap between naps. Little ones can often stay awake for around an hour longer at this time, but again, **this varies for each individual.**

So here are some examples:

Your baby may wake up in the morning between 7am and 7.30am. They may be able to handle being awake for 1.5 hours so they will go for a nap at around 8.30am if they woke at 7am, or they might not be ready to go for a nap until 9am if they woke up slightly later at 7.30am.

This is also true depending on the length of the naps.

So if your baby's first nap at 9am is 2 hours long and they wake up at 11am, then their next nap will be after they have been up for their 'awake time period' (for this example 1.5 hours) at 12.30pm. However if their first nap was only 45 minutes, then their second nap will be earlier at 11.15am.

> *During night feeds and night nappy changes, keep lights low and avoid too much talking and eye contact – just enough to keep them content without stimulating them*

I advise trying to have at least one of your little one's naps at home, in their bed. The others can be in the car or pram. If they tend to have a longer nap in the morning, then try to plan your activities and catch-ups for the afternoons when you can then get out and about.

Not all days will work out like this but if you can, try to make this the plan for the majority of the time.

CHAPTER 6 – WHY SLEEP TRAIN AT ALL?

The majority of babies need to learn or be taught how to fall asleep on their own.

'Sleep training' or teaching your baby to sleep can be a very emotional decision, wondering if you are doing the right thing by your baby.

But the key question to ask yourself is:

'Would I be a happier, healthier parent and would my baby be happier and healthier if we were both getting a good night's sleep?'

There are many parents out there who are completely against sleep teaching or training. They are more than happy to feed on demand throughout the day and night and have their little one rely on them to fall asleep. And this too is fine.

I often hear comments from parents against sleep training such as 'well my baby's not going to be 16 and still relying on me to fall asleep, I'll let her learn on her own in her own time'.

This type of thinking is all well and good if you are happy to always be with your baby and toddler.

For others (myself included) they feel trapped, claustrophobic and dislike the feeling of being constantly needed.

For me personally, and the many other mothers I interviewed, I wanted my freedom back, to at least have the choice to be able to go out with my friends in the evenings. To not have to worry about being home at a certain time to cuddle, rock, feed my little one to sleep.

When I had an event coming up that required me to be out in the evening, I would worry and stress for weeks in advance, thinking about how my little one was going to get to sleep without me. And worry also for the person looking after him, how would they cope?

Something needed to change.

My baby needed to learn to fall asleep without relying on mum or dad, and I needed my freedom back.

Parents need to feel in control, and while some sacrifice is certainly to be expected when becoming a parent, you need to be getting adequate sleep to remain sane.

Teaching a baby to sleep well early on in their lives, rather than letting them eventually learn on their own when they are potentially an older toddler, is definitely beneficial for both parents and baby.

For parents, the stress and complications that come along with lack of sleep can have devastating effects.

Marriages can breakdown. This is due to irritability and irrational behaviour. Too little sleep leaves you feeling emotional, unable to communicate effectively and patience wears very thin. Often petty arguments grow in to huge disagreements.

Mothers also have a higher chance of showing symptoms of depression when overtired. This in turn can affect bonding with babies.

Parents who aren't getting enough sleep are unable to be attentive and emotionally supportive to their little one, to help them through the huge mental and physical developments they are facing each day.

For babies, lack of sleep will also cause many of the same symptoms. Irritability, emotional, unable to concentrate, and unable to be attentive and adjust well to their developing world.

It has been proven that good sleep is vital for babies' learning and development. Babies that sleep well (especially at night) have higher mental and learning abilities – that's pretty major stuff!

Some sleep deprivation at times is to be expected during parenthood. **But** ongoing sleep deprivation can have serious effects.

So let's get this sleep issue sorted for the good of your whole family!

CHAPTER 7 – WHEN SHOULD MY BABY BE SLEEPING THROUGH THE NIGHT?

Well, this is a tricky one!

And the reason is (as I've mentioned a few times now) that every baby is different.

The age at which a baby first starts sleeping through the night depends on a few things:

Have they learnt how to fall asleep and resettle themselves during the night?

Some babies learn this skill relatively easily all on their own, but most need to be taught – cue **Baby Sleep Training In 3 Days** in the coming chapters

Are their bodies able to last 10-12 hours without a feed or drink?

This can come down to the amount of milk/food they are getting during the day.

And for breastfed babies it's not only to do with the baby's tummy being full enough to last the distance, but it also will depend greatly on the mother's milk supply and storage.

> *"People who say they sleep like a baby usually don't have one."*
> Leo J. Burke

This has no reflection on the size of the breasts – large breasts don't necessarily contain more milk. It is the storage capacity and the speed of milk production which can't be seen.

Some mothers have large storage and produce plenty of milk, only needing to feed their babies every 3-4 hours during the day providing enough to keep their little ones full all night.

Other mothers' breasts don't quite have this ability and physical storage in their breast and milk ducts and therefore need to feed more regularly, day and night.

The quality of the milk will make a difference too. If a breastfeeding mother isn't taking in enough calories to make good quality milk then the milk can be more 'watery' and not quite as filling. The content of the milk changes through the day also, with the fattiness changing as the day goes on.

And it's very normal to wonder if you are even making enough milk for your little one – we can't see how much babies are drinking from the breast so it can be a very hard one to gage.

If you suspect you aren't making enough milk and that your baby is draining the milk too quickly and is still hungry it is a good idea to get the opinion and help from a lactation consultant.

There are really great prescription and herbal remedies that you can take to improve your milk production and flow.

Wishing that your baby would sleep through the night isn't a good reason to switch from breastfeeding to formula though – this change can bring its own challenges. But at the same time, if you need to make this switch for whatever reason that is fine too.

Strangers, friends and family will all offer their opinions when it comes to feeding you baby, the same as they will for offering advice regarding your baby's sleep - take it all with a grain of salt and be confident in your decisions and ability.

Whatever age your baby is able to sleep through the night, does not necessarily mean that they will never wake in the night ever again (disappointing – right?!)

Even after your baby has reached the point where they *can* sleep through the night, it doesn't mean they *will* every single night.

Remember back to Section 1, Chapter 3, there are so many changes happening over these first few years that you need to be prepared for the odd bad night.

On average I would say that a baby is ready to sleep through the night at around 6 months old without needing a feed.

But that being said, some babies can do this much earlier, and others a little later.

And I know that this answer can be a little disappointing.

Try not to work towards a particular *age* at which your little one will sleep through the night, but focus more on their *ability* to sleep through the night.

The *ability* to fall asleep unassisted is the major part to this puzzle which can easily be learnt at any age.

The *ability* to last through the night without needing a feed will depend on the individual baby.

CHAPTER 8 – CRY IT OUT VS CONTROLLED COMFORTING

The Baby Sleep Training In 3 Days has options to cover each mother's opinions and values on whether or not it is ok to leave your baby to cry for **short** periods of time.

Numerous studies show that there is no long term harm in leaving your baby to cry for a limited time period, but there are also other studies that show that certain babies don't respond well to this and have an increased level of the stress hormone cortisol when left alone.

I often hear people referring to the Romanian orphanages when talking about the negative effects of leaving a young one to cry. They note that these orphanages are eerily quiet and the babies and children don't make a sound in their cribs. Implying that when these orphans are left to cry they soon learn and believe that there is no point crying out as no one will come to them.

I believe this is an extreme case, where these babies are not given a complete nurturing environment, they aren't happy and don't feel loved by their caregivers at anytime during the day or night, so they have begun to shut down emotionally.

If your baby is happy and healthy and you have a good loving, nurturing, caring home environment then leaving your baby for five minutes is completely acceptable and will not harm or have any long term negative effects.

I also believe and understand though that some parents find the thought of leaving their little ones alone for even this short amount of time simply too stressful. And if the parents aren't comfortable with the situation then the baby will certainly pick up on this uncertainty and may not react well.

It is after all a very natural instinct to rush to your baby when they cry.

You may find that in the night you wake a few seconds before your baby even makes a peep and begins to cry. We are designed this way as parents so it is certainly not an easy task to sit back and listen to the crying without rushing to their aid. I have some tips on how to help if you do choose this method.

I prefer to call it *'grizzle* it out' rather than *'cry* it out'. After the first night it will most likely be a grizzle as a protest rather than a scream or a cry.

Remember that you are changing the way you and your little one have been doing things so when they cry – being the only way they know how to communicate – this is simply their way of showing their frustration and confusion and this new situation.

As mentioned in Chapter 2 – You are the teacher, it is really important that you and your partner are in agreement with which method you wish to go with. You need to be a united front and be comfortable with your chosen method.

And stick to it!

You will choose whether you let your baby grizzle for limited time periods or stay close to them and gradually lead them in to sleep independence.

Remembering that leaving your baby alone for very short periods is the quicker method, but staying with them and supporting them through this change will also only take a few more nights and will still be effective.

Letting your baby 'cry it out' during The Sleep Training isn't about making your baby feel abandoned. This part was very important for me when I was creating this method. The amount of time we are giving them is enough for them to learn how to sleep, but not long enough for them to feel abandoned. You will still be regularly and periodically checking and verbally comforting your little one.

They will still love and adore you, I promise!

And if you choose to stay in the room with your little one, this is about gradually moving further away from them and slowing letting them know that you aren't far away and will always return.

The choice is yours, there is no right or wrong method. Choose whichever you are comfortable with.

> *"They eat, they crap, they sleep, and if they're crying they need to do one of the three and they're having trouble doing it. Real simple."*
>
> *Matthew McConaughey*

CHAPTER 9 – THE IMPORTANCE OF CONSISTENCY

I cannot stress enough how important being consistent is with babies and toddlers.

They thrive on routine and consistency. It is fine to change up your methods and try new things, however you need to stick to it.

Life is confusing enough for a little one. And even though they may protest, after a short time they will learn and expect what is coming.

This is true for both discipline and sleep training.

If you are trying to teach your baby or toddler not to hit for example, every single time they hit you should tell them no, and the reason why, and any consequences.

If you only follow this method *sometimes* they can get very confused – *it was ok to hit Dad on the arm before when we were play-wrestling, but now I'm getting growled at for hitting my little sister? I don't understand?.....*

> *Nicole was getting frustrated that her 20 month old toddler Simon repeatedly climbed up on to the bathroom sink, she was worried for his safety.*
>
> *Usually when she saw him climb up she would immediately pull him down and tell him that he could hurt himself. However, Nicole also knew that if he got up on the sink he was quiet and would play for 10 minutes on his own. With a newborn to look after as well, it was often tempting to leave him be and have 10 minutes peace and quiet.*
>
> *Poor Simon was confused when he was scolded for playing up on the sink one day, then left to play quietly the next.*

You can't expect them to learn what is acceptable or not if you aren't consistent.

So this is then also true for sleep training – *last night when I called out for Mum she came rushing in to pat me back to sleep, and earlier tonight she gently called to me from outside the bedroom door to reassure me, now she's ignoring me – what did I do wrong?....*

A lot of parents do struggle with consistency.

It can at times be difficult to be consistent if your baby is protesting slightly more than usual. It can simply be easier at times to give in. Knowing that if you just go in and rock them for a couple of minutes they will be asleep and you can get back to your evening.

Don't give in – be consistent!
Yes, it may be the slightly more difficult path to take today and for the next few days, but try to look to the future to once the skill or lesson has been learned.

Babies need time to learn and practice their new skill, in this instance we are talking about the skill of falling asleep on their own.

Babies and toddlers are very quick learners, look at how much they have learnt and achieved in such a small time period already! But they need the time and space to reinforce this.

It is also unfair on them to expect them to know what they should be doing when you keep changing things on them.

After a couple of nights you may be thinking that this sleep method isn't working for you.

I strongly suggest you stick at it and be consistent with it for a week. If you are committed to change this is the best strategy.

Consistency, consistency, consistency. And routine, routine, routine.

These words are so very important with babies and toddlers.

With the crucial bedtime **routines**, it is important to be **consistent.**

If you have a routine that goes something like this for example:
Bath – bottle – 2 books – cuddle & talk about the day – bed – sleep

It is important not to be talked in to adding in another book
Bath – bottle – 2 books – cuddle & talk about the day – bed – **book** – sleep

It's hard work taking care of little ones, and at the end of a long day it can be difficult to stick to your original plan. Or in the middle of the night, at the beginning of your sleep training when you have had a late night, and your baby has woken 20 minutes after you have fallen asleep yourself. But trust me, it will be worth it.

If you 'give in' one night because you can't bear the thought of a battle or a few tears, and you read the extra book, it is unfair for your little one to then accept that they can't have that extra book again the following night.

Being consistent is the fairest way to help your little one through this short, but possibly tough couple first days. And from there on in of course too.

If you swaddle your baby or use a grow-bag/sleeping-bag for your baby's sleeps, then make sure you use this for ALL naps and sleeps, not just night time. This soon becomes a signal to your little one that it is sleep time.

CHAPTER 10 – CRYING

A baby's cry is such a heart-breaking sound.

Parents, mothers especially, are programmed to respond to the sound of a baby's cry. It alerts our brain to kick in to gear and 'help our baby'.

And a lot of the time our baby does cry out for us when they need our help.

There are also other reasons babies cry though, and they don't necessarily need us to go rushing in to them at each and every peep they make.

A baby's cry is their only method of communication in the early months. It can be really tough going for both parents and babies before they learn to make other sounds to express themselves.

A baby may cry if they are bored, or want a change of scenery. If you have placed your baby on the ground with something to look at they may be happy playing there for 10 minutes then start to cry. They may simply be bored with whatever it is you have given them to look at, or they may need to be moved in to a different room or environment.

They may be uncomfortable with their position. You may have sat them up in a rocker or chair and they will seem to enjoy this position before they start slowly tipping over or are unable to control their head to sit up straight any longer.

Many babies enjoy the space and freedom of lying on a blanket on the ground instead. This gives them the ability to discover and move their limbs and bodies without straining their head and neck.

Babies (and older toddlers) like to know you are still there and close by. If you are out of their sight and they can't hear you they will cry out, thinking you have abandoned them. Try singing or talking to you little one while you are in the kitchen preparing dinner. It won't do them any harm by leaving them in a safe position for a few minutes to take a bathroom break, it is ok to let them express that they are missing you through crying out to you. If you are uncomfortable with this then distraction is a wonderful thing – turn the TV on or a musical toy to distract them for a few minutes.

Some babies are particularly fussy about having a wet or dirty nappy and will let you know about it! My baby boy wasn't bothered at all by a dirty nappy, but my little girl cried out instantly when she was requesting a nappy change.

Most babies also really love the freedom of having a kick around on the ground with no nappy on. It is really important to give them as much 'nappy free' time as possible as this also allows them to move more freely and explore their bodies more easily.

Babies let us know when they are hungry by crying out. But they may also cry out for 'hunger' as a means of comfort.

There is nothing wrong with breast feeding your baby for comfort as well as hunger. Often babies will just suck without taking on a lot of milk. If this is too demanding on you as the breastfeeding mom, then a pacifier can sometimes be a good alternative. The sucking motion is such a comfort for little babies especially.

> *Louise's little girl Sophie would cry at each feed when she would talk or when there were people close by who were talking. Once Louise figured out that the noise was what was upsetting and distracting Sophie, she began going to a quieter room for feeds (not easy with a toddler in the house!) She slowly started feeding with the TV or radio on and starting turning up the volume from very quiet and increasing it to get Sophie used to having more noise around.*

Some babies are more prone to wind or gas than others. It can be very uncomfortable for babies unable to bring up their wind and they may need your help to do so.

During or after each feed, bring your baby upright.

You could try resting their head on your shoulder and patting their back to release the wind. Another method is to sit them on your knee with your palm on their chest and their head and neck resting on between your thumb and pointer finger, then pat their back with your other hand.

One of my favourite winding techniques I call the **Merry-go-Round Technique.**

To use this method, sit baby on your knee, with one hand on their chest

(as in the above technique) and place your other hand on their back. Slowly move the baby in a circular motion in one direction making a circle four times, and then repeat in the other direction. This helps 'loosen' the wind and you can then give a couple of gentle pats on the back to help bring it right up if needed.

Some babies are bothered by little things such as a sock that has a piece of cotton pulling on their little toe, by a clothing label tag scratching their neck or by a pair of pants that are slightly too tight on their waist.

Sometimes a little piece of Mom's hair could be tangled around their finger annoying them.

Check for all of these things and that they aren't too hot or cold. Babies often have cool or clammy hands and feet, but this doesn't mean they are cold. To check this, place your hand down their back and check to see if they are sweaty or feel cool.

Some more sensitive babies are simply overwhelmed by the world around them.

Noise, colour, people can all be too much sometimes.

Often babies cry and parents pick them up, walk around, sing and try every trick they know to stop the crying, when all the baby really wants is to be put on the floor and given some space.

Try some soothing classical music, such as 'Brahms Lullaby'.

And babies of course cry when they are getting tired.

It can often be a bit of a guessing game trying to figure out what the crying is all about.

Each baby is sensitive to different things and will cry for different reasons, so try these different techniques and learn what your baby wants and dislikes.

Neither of my babies enjoyed being around lots of people until they were about 6 months old. Those first 6 months I felt quite claustrophobic, and alone, but I slowly introduced them to different environments with a few more people and I now have one very social child and one who is more shy.

It is important to remember to do what works best for you and your baby, not what other parents and babies do.

CHAPTER 11 – BABY SLEEP POSITIONS

It is always recommended to place your baby on their back to sleep.

These recommendations come from The American Academy of Paediatrics, The World Health Organisations and other highly credible associations.

For the first couple of months of a baby's life this is especially important.

A baby sleeping on their stomach can potentially have an increased chance of suffering from SIDS (Sudden Infant Death Syndrome). This is all very scary and the thoughts around this are still being researched; however the thinking is that a baby sleeping on their front will possibly breathe less effectively.

After the first few months of your baby's life, if they enjoy sleeping on their back then continue this, sleeping on their back is the safest position.

But, as we have already discovered, not all babies are created equal. There is no *normal* when it comes to babies. Some babies simply don't enjoy the position of sleeping on their back. I know for me personally, I can't sleep lying flat on my back.

There is no specific age at when it is ok to change the sleep position. Just like there is no specific age at when you should introduce a bottle, or a pacifier, or to begin sleep teaching.

> *Don't sleep babies with a hat on, they need to regulate their body temperature and can't do this if their head is covered. Try instead to heat the room or add an additional layer of clothing or blankets*

Use your parental instincts and do what works best for you, your baby and your family. Just because your neighbour, friend or mother tells you they did something one way at a particular age does not mean that this is right for you and your little one.

If you are wanting to place your baby on their side or front to sleep, please ensure you consult your baby's doctor or childcare provider first.

If your baby is able to roll, then they may turn themselves on to their side or back on their own, of course you can't be there all night to watch and flip them back over when this occurs! If they are at this stage in their development, and they enjoy sleeping on their front then I don't see the harm in placing them in to bed in this position.

The key thing to safety in this position is that the baby is able to lift and move their head to clear the way for breathing.

Before placing your baby to sleep in any position, there are a few things you can do to make the environment safer:

- Use a firm mattress.

- Avoid placing babies on soft surfaces such pillows or quilts.

- Don't use infant sleep positioners which often use Velcro to hold a baby in a certain position.

- If your baby can roll, or if you are placing them in bed on their side or front, do not swaddle.

- Avoid placing soft toys at the top of the bed, or in the bed at all.

- Keep pets out of the sleeping baby's room.

Using a bassinette for the first weeks or months of a baby's life is a good idea but not a necessity.

It can just be another expense at a very costly time – these babies aren't cheap to run!

And depending on how big your baby is when they are born, and how quickly they grow, it could be only used for a matter of weeks before they are too big for it.

A bassinette is smaller and therefore a new, small baby can feel more secure in there.

An alternative option is to put your baby straight in to a cot or crib. These are much larger and can be used for a few years.

It is a good idea to invest in a new and good quality mattress. When you look at how much time your little one will be spending in there it makes sense to ensure it is clean, comfortable and firm. Many people purchase the outer part of the crib second-hand and spend the money on a new mattress. If you are purchasing any part second hand, always ensure it has come from a smoke-free and pet-free environment if possible.

My feelings on co-sleeping with your baby are that it should be avoided where possible.

This isn't to do with the fact that there are added dangers in doing this (the possibility of rolling on to your little one, or suffocating with the larger blankets etc on an adult's bed)

My reason for wanting to avoid this is so that you all can get a better night's sleep.

Sure, some women like to be able to easily roll over and breastfeed their baby really having to move much, this can make things easier. However if your baby stirs and is left for a minute or two they may fall back to sleep on their own. If you don't give them this opportunity and immediately feed them instead, this will then begin to be expected and so begins a cycle of many more night feedings than required – and who wants more night wake ups than necessary?!

Plus – babies can be noisy little sleepers! You won't sleep deeply with a snuffly loud baby on you or close by. And a well rested parent equals a much happier family.

CHAPTER 12 – SLEEP PROPS AND ASSOCIATIONS

Sleep Props and Associations are things that your little one relies on to fall asleep.

When babies are newborn we try anything in those early weeks to get them to sleep.

We rock and cuddle them – who can resist a newborn snuggling in to their chest as they sleep – watching their fascinating facial movements and eyelid flutters, bliss!

We jiggle them, we give them a pacifier to suck on. We swaddle them and sing or hum a gentle lullaby.

We also sometimes invest a lot of money on gadgets promising to assist with our baby falling asleep, I know I did!

However, some sleep props and associations begin to be bad habits, while others are important to the sleep process.

For example, a bedtime routine is a Sleep Association, but it is an important cue to your little one that bedtime is approaching, a wind down period – *when done correctly.*

Snugglies, favourite soft toys or Blankies are a Sleep Prop, but can also be a Sleep Association if you only give them to your baby at sleep times.

> *If your little one has a snugly, favourite soft toy or blankie, get a duplicate to avoid a disaster if one is lost or left somewhere. Switch them out regularly so they wear and smell the same.*

Sleep Props such as White Noise, Pacifiers and Movement are all great to help calm your baby and keep them asleep, but having to rely on these can cause major issues when your baby needs these again and again during the night and you are having to get up over and over again to jiggle them back to sleep or replace a pacifier.

If your baby is still relying on the sleep props, there are some easy ways to remove *some of these*, others are important to **keep.**

Now that you know that your little one doesn't need you to rock them to sleep or lull them in to a deep slumber, they also don't *need* to rely on some of these Sleep Props and Associations either.

White noise

When babies are in the uterus they are surrounded by constant and very loud noise. When I say loud, it is thought to be about as loud as standing directly under a running shower or near a lawnmower!

Babies are used to loudly hearing their mother's heart beating, breathing, blood flowing and the muffling sound of mommy's voice. So coming out in to the world and being placed in a bed in a quiet room is very unusual and unsettling to begin with.

Babies enjoy a constant sound – loud bangs and other sudden noises can also be unsettling and frightening for them.

You may notice that your baby falls asleep easily in the car – this is because of the car engine noise (along with the movement and vibrations) or at the mall – where there is a constant hum and chatter.

'Shhhhuuuusssssshhhhhh-ing' your baby is somewhat of a natural instinct of a noise that parents use to calm their baby. This is a form of White Noise also that you can make yourself. You'll notice that the louder you 'shush' the quicker your baby begins to calm down.

White Noise is a constant and repetitive sound. Some parents play talkback radio, others play classical music. Just finding static on the radio and playing this also works. There are many devices, toys and music tracks that play womb-like sounds also – a loud, low pitched noise, similar to a vacuum cleaner with a pulsating rhythm.

It works by blocking out other stimulation – this is pretty much everything going on around your baby, lights, faces, images.

Calming noises like rain fall work particularly well also.

These sounds played loudly can help to calm an upset baby; play the noise as your baby is falling asleep and it will help lull them to sleep.

White Noise also can help with blocking out daily sounds such as a father getting up early in the morning to go to work, or the rubbish truck on the street outside, or the neighbour's car horn.

This issue with this, as well as other sleep props, is that when your baby partially wakes in the night they may then need the noise once again to drift in to the next sleep cycle.

If you have started using White Noise and want to phase it out, there is an easy way to remove it using my Dimmer Method.

Simply turn down the volume on whatever it is you are playing slightly more each day over a five day period, until the sound is so low you can remove it all together.

Pacifier/Dummy

The sucking motions that a baby uses when breast or bottle feeding are also particularly soothing for a baby. Babies are born with the need to suck, it is a natural reflex that they rely to survive, as well as soothe.

Some breastfeeding mothers love any opportunity to feed their little one, while others feel smothered and like they are constantly pinned down to the couch with a baby attached to them. You see, babies want to feed for thirst and hunger, *but also for comfort.* Pacifiers can be a God-send for some parents. It can give you a break from comfort feeding and constant holding.

Some dentists recommend removing the pacifier before the age of 4 to avoid dental issues.
In my experience though, it is best to remove it much earlier that this - but, as with many issues to do with babies and toddlers, there are many varying opinions on what *is* the correct or best age.

If your little one is crying out in the night to have it replaced, or if you think they are relying on it too much and they are beginning to speak with it in, then it is a good time to look at removing it altogether.

There are a couple of ways to go about removing Pacifiers.

Go cold turkey – that is to take the pacifier away one day and don't ever give it back! It sounds harsh but this is the fastest way to eliminate it.

If your toddler is old enough, get them to take the pacifier (along with any other spares you have in the house) and put them in the rubbish bin. Talk to them about why they don't need it so that when it comes to sleep time or in the night you can remind them about your conversation.

If you are going to go with this method, as with most things to do with babies and toddlers **be consistent.**

This may be one of those times you need to use **The Baby Sleep Training Method** *Refresher.*

Don't have any *backups or spares* kept aside in case you have a rough night during the removal process, you may well be tempted to give in if you have them there.

If you don't think the cold turkey method is for you, here is a little trick I learnt and tried and it worked really well! It is called **The Haircut Method.**

The Haircut Method works like this - trim a small amount off the end of the pacifier and give it to your little one as usual. With the tip removed it will make the sucking motion they enjoy slightly trickier. Each day over the next five days trim slightly more off until there is nothing left to suck.

They will lose interest pretty quickly – simple!

Swaddle

Swaddling your baby is where you wrap them firmly. The reason newborns like and need to be swaddled is that it limits their movements, particularly their arm movements. They feel much more calm and relaxed when they feel safe and secure.

Think about when they were in the womb, as they grew they had very little room to move, a feeling like they were held safe. Swaddling recreates this feeling.

Babies are born with a startle reflex where their arms and legs flail and appear to jump or move suddenly. They have no control of their limbs in these early days – in fact they don't even know that those limbs are even theirs yet!

It is best to limit swaddling to sleep time only, or those times where they are particularly unsettled as a means to calm them down. It is important to limit it to these times only as it is equally as important for babies to stretch out and begin to learn and discover their new little bodies.

I think it is really important to swaddle your baby for the first few months, until they are close to rolling – at this point it is best to remove the swaddle so that if they roll on to their front they have their arms free to help push their head up or move back in to a safer position.

When it does come time to remove the swaddle, I find it best to remove it by using **The Ladder Technique**

The Ladder Technique works like this –

Day One: Swaddle slightly looser than usual, but still holding the arms in, high and near the body.

Day Two: Swaddle as on Day One, but this time leave one arm up, out of the swaddle.

Day Three: Swaddle as on Day One, but this time switch the arm so that the opposite arm is left out and up and one is still in the swaddle. Day Four: Swaddle the body and leave both of the arms out, your baby will naturally put their arms up.

Day Five: Remove the Swaddle altogether.

Routines

I have mentioned a few times now in this book how important consistency and routines are.

Taking in to account the above when we are looking at removing some Sleep Props and Associations, it is really important to keep the Sleep Association of **Routine.**

We want to ensure our little ones still know it is sleep time, we want them to feel confident and comfortable with what is going on.

Now I know that Routines can very easily be draaaaaagggggged out but smart little babies and toddlers, adding another book, song or milk request.

No matter the age of your little one, stick to your routine, and be consistent.

Here is a good example of a Routine:

Food
Wind down time with quiet play
Bath or Shower
Breast or bottle feed
One Book
Bed

This Routine works for night time, but naps should be fairly similar, with the bath or shower removed.

Put a Routine in place and stick to it every night.

On those nights were you are going out and having a sitter look after your little one (now that you have completed **The Baby Sleep Training** programme you will have so much more energy and will feel like getting out and about socialising again) make sure that you go through the routine with the caregiver and ask them to be firm with this also.

If you are going out for the evening, taking the little one with you and planning on being home a bit later, you can still complete the routine, just take out the bath/shower and go with breast or bottle feed, one book then bed.

It is important to remember that babies and children can work around appointment and important events, not every day or night will fit in to your routine. Just try to keep your routine the majority of the time. Be as *consistent as possible*.

CHAPTER 13 – THE FIVE MINUTE SLEEP METHOD

The Five Minute Sleep Method is the one and only method I have found that works, by allowing the baby time to learn the all-important skill of falling asleep.

You are also teaching them that you are there for them and are not abandoning them.

Falling asleep on their own is likely the only way they will then be able to drift back to sleep in the night in between sleep cycles.

Many 'sleep training' methods encourage you to leave you baby to cry for increased periods of time, even up to 30 minutes or more of crying alone, I have read one method suggesting you walk away and don't come back until the morning! This makes me really sad for the baby, and the parents that have though that this is the best or only option.

The Five Minute Sleep Method is all about letting your little one know that you aren't far away, that you will *always return to help them*, and that they can fall asleep without being fed, held or rocked.

My trials of this method showed me that the time of five

minutes was the perfect amount of time for babies to learn how to fall asleep on their own, but not long enough to feel abandoned.

I also found that increasing this time period over the evening doesn't help at all, in fact I think that this is just confusing for them.

I suggest you start this programme with a night time sleep, and then continue it on to the following days naps and then night again.

Before you start, ensure that the timing is right. By this I mean, ensure that your little one is healthy, don't start when they have a cold or a temperature (even though it is during these times that their sleeping is often at it's worst) Don't choose the night after immunisations or if they have had a particularly unsettled day for whatever reason.

Also, ensure that you are in the right frame of mind. Be confident in your ability to teach your baby. And as mentioned earlier, make sure that all caregivers present are on board.

Here is a simple checklist before you start:
My baby is healthy
My partner and I are both committed to using this program every day and night for up to one to two weeks
My baby is tired and ready for sleep

1ST NIGHT

Step One

Firstly, decide whether you are going to stay with your little one in the room throughout the process of falling asleep, or whether you are comfortable to leave them on their own to learn this skill, remember – you will be checking on them regularly.

Step Two:

Once you have set up routines for both naps and bedtime you are ready to start teaching your baby how to fall asleep on their own, and this in turn will lead to teaching them how to stay asleep without fully waking in between sleep cycles.

Ensure your baby is fed (and winded if they are still in their early months) and clean, then complete your bedtime routine, and place your baby safely in bed.

Step Three

Tell your little one that it is sleep time and give them a comforting, reassuring rub on the tummy or back.

Night one will be the hardest, once this is complete it gets much easier the next couple of nights then the battle will be over!

Step Four - If you have decided to leave your baby for a short period of time:

Walk out of the room, while reassuring your little one. Say something like 'night night, time for sleep, I love you'

Leave your baby for **Five Minutes.**

Make sure to use a stop watch or clock of some sort, I can guarantee that it will seem longer than it really is. A distraction can be good, wash the dishes, or fold some laundry, anything to help the short time pass even more quickly.

Step Four - If you have decided to stay in the room with your baby:

Have a chair positioned next to the baby's bed.

Reassure your little one. Say something like 'night night, time for sleep, I love you'

Sit on the chair for **Five Minutes***. Make sure to use a stop watch or clock of some sort, I can guarantee that it will seem longer than it really is.*

Do not say anything more to your baby, and don't get up to them - just being near them will be enough. If your baby and you are getting distressed you can offer a reassuring 'ssshhhhhh, mom's here' only.

Step Five - If you have decided to leave your baby for a short period of time:

Once the time is up, if your baby is crying, return to them and repeat the process of telling your little one that it is sleep time – repeat the phrase you used in Step Three, don't say anything more than that and give them a quick reassuring rub on the tummy or back. This process should be less than one minute. Walk out of the room and leave them for **Five Minutes** *once again. Repeat until your baby is asleep.*

If your baby is awake but not crying, leave them on their own even after the time is up.

If they stop crying during the five minutes, then start again, start timing another five minutes from when they started again.

Step Five – If you have decided to stay in the room with your baby

Once the time is up, if your baby is still awake, stand up, go to your little one and repeat the process of telling your little one that it is sleep time – repeat the phrase you used in Step Three. Don't say anything more than that and give them a quick reassuring rub on the tummy or back.

Sit back on your chair next to the crib and leave them for **Five Minutes** *once again.*

If they stop crying during the five minutes, then start again, start timing another five minutes from when they started again.

This first night is the hardest, it will get easier from here on in, and in a few nights time you will be completing your bedtime routine, placing baby in their crib and not returning until the morning – bliss!

Once your baby is asleep, they may wake in the night still. If your baby is over 6 months old and you and your baby's health care professionals are comfortable that they don't need extra feeds during the night then repeat the steps above.

For the first night in particular, it can be a good idea to stay close to the baby's room to listen out for any signs of real distress. If they have had a breast feed or bottle immediately before being placed in to bed then some babies may get worked up enough to spill up their milk.

Step One

Firstly, decide whether you are going to stay with your little one in the room throughout the process of falling asleep, or whether you are comfortable to leave them on their own to learn this skill, remember – you will be checking on them regularly.

2nd DAY & NIGHT ONWARDS

If you have decided to leave your baby for a short period of time:

Repeat the process of Night One.

If you have decided to stay in the room with your baby:

Repeat the process of Night One, however move the chair that you are sitting on in the room slightly closer to the door.

As each night passes, the chair should be positioned closer and closer to the door, until you are sitting outside of the room.

At this stage if you need to then you can use Steps Three and Four from 'If you have decided to leave your baby for a short period of time.'

Wake Ups During the Night:

If your baby is under 6 months and you feel like they should need a feed during a waking in the night then quietly pick them up, don't chatter with them, keep the room dark and quiet.

Return them to their bed and repeat the steps above.

After a few nights, perhaps slightly longer if you have used the 'Stay in the room with your baby' method, your baby will have learnt how to fall asleep without your assistance, and they will be assured and comfortable that you are close by, and will return to them when they need you.

Congratulations for sticking to the method and achieving your goal – **SUCCESS**!!!!

As mentioned in Chapter Three, there may be bumps along the road going forward, but take comfort in knowing that your little one has just learnt a truly valuable life skill, and that your lives are getting back on track.

> *The optimum room temperature for sleep is between 65 and 70 degrees Fahrenheit, and between 18 and 21 degrees Celsius*

CHAPTER 14 – THE FIVE MINUTE SLEEP METHOD REFRESHER

Once you have completed the Five Minute Sleep Method training successfully you may be thinking that you will never be woken in the night again, or never have any issues getting your baby or toddler to sleep.

Unfortunately, parenting is never that simple.

There will be times when your little one may regress from their fantastic sleeping.

Examples of this could be when they are unwell, teething, having a growth spurt, going through a mental or developmental change.

Believe me when I reassure you that parents who say their baby sleeps through the night *every single night* are simply exaggerating. I would say this is nearly impossible for a baby to do.

It can be a relatively quick process to what seems like 'undoing' all your hard work from the initial Sleep training. But rest assured, it is also a very quick process to get back on track.

I have mentioned earlier that five minutes is the optimal time period to leave your baby to learn how to fall asleep on their own whilst still knowing that you are not abandoning them. In the refresher below, you will see that we do leave them for 10 minutes after the initial period of 5 minutes, but they have already learnt the skill - we are simply reminding them.

By this stage they know and trust that you are there for them. If however, you aren't comfortable with this time period you can stick to the 5 minutes with no problems at all, other than the process may take an extra night or so.

This is the basic formula on how the Five Minute Sleep Method **REFRESHER** works:

1st NIGHT

Step One:

Decide again whether you are going to stay with your little on in the room throughout the process of falling asleep, or whether you are comfortable to leave them on their own to learn this skill, checking on them regularly.

Step Two:

Complete your bedtime routine, and then place your baby safely in bed.

Step Three

Tell your little one that it is sleep time and give them a comforting, reassuring rub on the tummy or back.

Remember again - night one will be the hardest, once this is complete it gets much easier the next couple of nights then the battle will be over!

Step Four - If you have decided to leave your baby for a short period of time:

Walk out of the room, while reassuring your little one. Say something like 'night night, time for sleep, I love you' Leave your baby for **Five Minutes**.

Make sure to use a stop watch or clock of some sort, I can guarantee that it will seem longer than it really is. A distraction can be good, wash the dishes, or fold some laundry, anything to help the short time pass even more quickly.

Step Four - If you have decided to stay in the room with your baby:

Have a chair positioned next to the baby's bed.

Reassure your little one. Say something like 'night night, time for sleep, I love you' Sit on the chair for **Five** *Minutes. Make sure to use a stop watch or clock of some sort, I can guarantee that it will seem longer than it really is.*

Do not say anything more to your baby, and don't get up to them - just being near them will be enough. If your baby and you are getting distressed you can offer a reassuring 'ssshhhhh' only.

Step Five - If you have decided to leave your baby for a short period of time:

Once the time is up, if your baby is crying, return to them and repeat the process of telling your little one that it is sleep time – repeat the phrase you used in Step Three, don't say anything more than that and give them a quick reassuring rub on the tummy or back.

*Walk out of the room and leave them for **TEN** Minutes.*

Repeat until your baby is asleep (only increase the time period by 5 Minutes ONCE.)

If your baby is awake but not crying, leave them on their own even after the time is up.

Step Five – If you have decided to stay in the room with your baby

Once the time is up, if your baby is still awake, stand up, go to your little one and repeat the process of telling your little one that it is sleep time – repeat the phrase you used in Step Three. Don't say anything more than that and give them a quick reassuring rub on the tummy or back.

*Sit back on your chair next to the crib and leave them for **TEN** minutes.*

Repeat until your baby is asleep (only increase the time period by 5 Minutes ONCE.) Keep to this increased time period until your little one is asleep.

If your baby is awake but not crying, leave them on their own even after the time is up.

As before, this first night is the hardest, it will get easier from here on in, and in a few nights time you will be completing your bedtime routine, placing baby in their crib and not returning until the morning – bliss once again!

Once your baby is asleep, they may wake in the night still. If your baby is over 6 months old and you and your baby's health care professionals are comfortable that they don't need extra feeds during the night then repeat the steps above.

If your baby is under 6 months and you feel like they should need a feed during a waking in the night then quietly pick them up, don't chatter with them, keep the room dark and quiet.
Return them to their bed and repeat the steps above.

2ND DAY & NIGHT ONWARDS:

> **If you have decided to leave your baby for a short period of time:**
>
> *Repeat the process of Night One.*

> **Night Two onwards:**
>
> **If you have decided to stay in the room with your baby:**
>
> *Repeat the process of Night One, however move the chair that you are sitting on in the room slightly closer to the door. As each night passes, the chair should be positioned closer and to the door, until you are sitting outside of the room. At this stage if you need to then you can use Steps Three and Four from* **If you have decided to leave your baby for a short period of time.**

After only a couple of nights, your baby will have remembered and re-learnt how to fall asleep without your assistance, and they will be assured and comfortable that you are close by, and will return to them when they need you.

Congratulations for sticking to the method once again and achieving your goal – **SUCCESS**!!!!

SECTION 2

CHAPTER 1 – MEDICAL CONDITIONS - REFLUX

It is important to rule out any medical issues your baby may have as to the cause of being unsettled.

Many parents want to find a reason that their baby won't sleep. They want to find a quick fix or a diagnosis with a medication to 'cure' the sleep issue. Every now and again though, there can be medical reason that is preventing your child from being relaxed enough to sleep well.

It is really important to trust your instincts but also trust the medical professionals.

Always, always seek medical advice if you are unsure or think your little one may be suffering from a medical issue.

There are a few medical conditions that could be affecting your baby or toddler's sleep including reflux.

When babies are born it is common for the valve in between the food pipe from the mouth and the stomach not to be fully formed, this can cause the milk along with stomach acids to be brought up and the baby spills or vomits.

Some 'spilly' babies are not bothered at all by the vomiting, however some others find it very painful, especially from the stomach acid causing a burning sensation for them.

Reflux can affect both breast fed and bottle fed babies.

Even babies without reflux will spill often. Remember that their stomachs are tiny when they are newborn, so their little tummies can't hold too much. Sometimes they simply take too much milk on board and their stomachs can't handle the volume.

Over time, this valve becomes stronger and the stomach size increases. They are able to cope with keeping the milk and stomach acid down and this in turn keeps the baby much happier.

If you suspect your baby has reflux you can try very slightly propping up their bassinette or crib, by only an inch or two. Having them on a very slight angle can really help with keeping the stomach acid down and decrease the burning sensation.

Try using a folded up towel under the mattress at the top of the basinet or crib.

Or put a thin book under the top two legs to raise the head up slightly.

> *Angela and Michael couldn't figure out why their 2 month old Blake would easily fall asleep on their shoulder, or in a bouncer but would wake within minutes of being put down in to his bassinet he would wake screaming. Blake didn't even need to be rocked or bounced to sleep but would only sleep in these positions.*
>
> *Their doctor suggested that they prop up his bassinet. They folded a towel up, placed it under his mattress at the top of the bed and immediately noticed a change in their little boy who went from only sleeping on them to be able to sleep in his bassinet.*
>
> *At 5 months old they noticed Blake was much more settled so tried unfolding the towel gradually to see if Blake could cope with a slightly flatter surface. He managed well and they were able to remove the towel all together within another week.*

Many mothers will have suffered reflux during pregnancy so will be able to relate to the discomfort.

If nothing seems to help the pain and discomfort of reflux, ensure you see your medical professional. In extreme cases, once a few tests have been performed a doctor may need to prescribe an anti-reflux medication to assist with comfort.

> *Dress your baby in natural materials only, 100% cotton for a base layer and wool over the top if it is particularly cold. Blankets should follow the same rule. Avoid polyester and polar fleece materials as they can prevent the skin from 'breathing' and cause sweating.*

CHAPTER 2 – SEPARATION ANXIETY

Babies, Toddlers and Children always need their parents (adults do too!)

When babies are newborn they will often go to strangers, are happy to be passed around as long as their needs are met.

At around 5-8 months babies reach a developmental milestone where they become aware that their parent or caregiver is not near them, or that a stranger is now holding them.

Separation anxiety is when a baby or toddler becomes stressed or anxious when a caregiver (often the mother if she is the one doing most of the feeding and caretaking) leaves. This can be when they leave for work for the day, or even just leave to go to the bathroom.

It is a trait that is developed very early on, a survival method, recognising that they rely on their parents to provide life for them, and that a stranger is a potential threat. They cry (or scream!) out for rescuing, to help them.

It's nice to feel needed and wanted, but it can also feel very claustrophobic and draining, unable to even place your child down while you prepare the dinner is very tiring!

Separation anxiety can continue right through to toddlerhood – that's a long time to constantly hold and be near your baby.

During these times try to think of the positive points – your little one loves and needs you, you have done a fantastic job of bonding with your baby, you are their world!

If you have other children that also need your attention during these times, or if you physically need a break then verbal reassurance can help. Talk or sing to your little one so they can hear your voice, this lets them know of your presence.

Remember also that little ones pick up on the feelings and vibe of the people around them so try to remain calm. It can be frustrating having a baby that is constantly crying, whinging or seemingly unhappy. Even though it may seem that nothing you are doing is helping them, just being near them will be helping.

Baby wearing is fantastic during these times also. Put your baby in a sling or baby wrap and it is much easier to carry on with your day, you can get out and about or just do your chores while they are close to you.

Babies and toddlers who are experiencing separation anxiety can once again begin waking at night; they want to be reassured that you are still there. You are their everything right now so it's a scary thought for them that you might not be coming back, that they are all alone.

During this time you may need to run through **The Five Minute Sleep Method Refresher.** This method is particularly helpful as you are constantly going back in to them to reassure them that they are safe and they you are still near.

Some babies experience separation anxiety to more extreme measures than others. If you have had a particularly unsettled baby from early on then these babies can be more sensitive, these feelings can be more heightened.

Having a baby going through separation anxiety, no matter how small or extreme the case may be, can be a fairly frustrating and tiring time – but try to remember what it is happening in your baby's world, so much is changing and they are coping with so much. All they want is to feel safe and secure.

CHAPTER 3 – ELIMINATING EARLY MORNING WAKINGS AND LATE NIGHT BEDTIMES

Just like adults, some babies are night owls, others are early risers.

It can be the luck of the draw as to whether your baby falls in to one of these categories or not...... but there are are few simple things you can do to eliminate these issues if they don't fit in to your schedule.

Many websites and books out there have very confusing and conflicting advice on these issues, such as *'Don't put your baby to bed to early'* and *'Make sure your baby isn't going to bed too late'*, *'Don't let them get overtired'* and *'Ensure they're tired enough to sleep 12 hours'*. *'Make sure they are having good naps and getting enough sleep during the day'* and *'Don't let them sleep too long at nap times during the day or they won't need enough sleep at night'*

How confusing!

My method and tips are much simpler.

As I talked about earlier with **The Gap Effect** in Section 1, Chapter 5, it can be hard to get it right with timings. I tend to focus on time period your little one can handle being awake for between naps. This gap between naps and bedtime is important, and should be reasonably stable, with the gap stretching slightly more as the months and years go by.

Early Morning Wakings

If you have a baby who is rising each morning at 6am or even 5am(!) this can be very tiring. I always like to get up at around 7am, half an hour before my babies wake at 7.30am (the majority of the time) so that I can enjoy my breakfast and have a quick shower in peace.

This didn't use to be the case however when my babies were waking at 6.30am, I simply couldn't drag myself out of bed at 6am – I am not a morning person!

Some factors such as illness or teething can create a temporary problem with early waking. If it is continuing then it has become a pattern, or the 'normal'.

If your baby is waking at 6.30am, is happy, in a good mood and not needing a nap to catch-up on the missed sleep from the early hours then this might not be an issue at all. Or is a 6am wakeup fits in with your schedule then that's great too!

BUT, babies who wake early, often then have a nap an hour or two later. They need this nap to get them through the morning or day as they have been up since the crack of dawn! This nap however is a big part of the early morning wakeup problem.

Babies' bodies think of this nap soon after waking as an extension of bedtime. They woke up at 6am, back down at 7am, then up again at 8am. Their brains are only counting the 8am wake up as the start of the day.

To start with, treat any waking **before 6am as a night waking.** That is, do the same thing at 5am as you would at 1.30am. Tuck them back in. Don't get them up until **6am at the very earliest.** Keep the room dark until this time, and only whisper – just as you would in the middle of the night.

Next, we need to set the body clock again. We can do this using my **Five Day Early Wake Method.**

Day One: Start their first nap of the day 15 minutes later than usual Day Two: Start their first nap of the day 15 minutes later than usual Day Three: Start their first nap of the day 30 minutes later than usual Day Four: Start their first nap of the day 45 minutes later than usual Day Five: Start their first nap of the day 1 hour later than usual

Say for example your little one is waking at 6am, and they are needing their first nap at 7.30am:

Day One: Start their first nap of the day at 7.45am
Day Two: Start their first nap of the day at 7.45am
Day Three: Start their first nap of the day at 8am
Day Four: Start their first nap of the day at 8.15am
Day Five: Start their first nap of the day at 8.30am

You should notice that by dragging out the early morning nap time, the morning wake time is also naturally dragged out.

> *Use a warm wet cloth to wipe baby's bottom instead of a packet wet wipe to avoid a cold shock, especially at night changes*

Late Night Bedtimes

While I was pregnant with my second child I was tired by the time the evening finally came around. I was working and looking after a toddler, as well as growing another human being – exhausting!

My toddler wasn't going to bed until 8.30pm and wasn't asleep until at least 9pm at the very earliest. I was having to wait up for him to go to sleep before I could get myself to bed!

I needed to get him to bed earlier. He was also sleeping late in the morning and I was having to wake him up to go to work.

I considered dropping his day nap – he was only having one. But I knew that he needed this (I needed him to have it too!).

This is where **The Sleep Gap System** from Section 1, Chapter 5 is really helpful.

If your little one is not falling asleep until late at night, you need to bring the wakeup time of the last nap back.

The best way to do this is do it gradually, using the Five Day Last Nap Gap Method.

For example, if your little one is waking up from their last nap at 4pm, and not going to sleep at night until 8pm, then you need to wake them earlier from that last nap.

Day 1 : Wake your little on 10 minutes earlier than usual
Day 2 : Wake your little on 15 minutes earlier than usual
Day 3 : Wake your little on 20 minutes earlier than usual
Day 4 : Wake your little on 25 minutes earlier than usual
Day 5 : Wake your little on 30 minutes earlier than usual

By now, your little one should be ready for bed at 7.30pm rather than 8pm.

> *It's not unusual for a newborn not to settle down for the night until around 9pm. This means that a 6.30pm-7pm sleep is their last nap for the day (often a short 'catnap') This can last for the first few months until they are around 4 months old*

CHAPTER 4 – DROPPING NAPS

How do you know when it is time to drop a nap from your baby or toddler?

After about three months of age, your baby should be somewhat predictable as to the number of naps they are having. The time they have their naps and the length of the nap may be changeable – try not to get too caught up on a strict time schedule eg. *'It's 12.15pm so my baby should be down for her 2nd nap of the day now.'* Try instead to focus on the gap between the naps eg *'My baby has been awake for 2 hours so it's time for her to go back to bed now.'*

As they get older, this gap between naps becomes longer and therefore naturally the number of naps decreases.

Naps become a battle and your baby or toddler starts resisting them, rather than taking 10-20 minutes to fall asleep, they start whinging for an hour or so before they finally start their nap.

If you are lucky enough to have a little one who has long naps (over 1.5 hours) then your baby will generally be ready to drop a nap earlier that a baby who only naps for 45 minutes at a time.

Some days are simply 'blowout days' where the naps are all over the show, you have been out and the little one fell asleep for 4 minutes in the car just before you made it home and they have woken up deciding that is enough sleep for them.

This will happen every now and again and while these days are horrendous and nothing goes to plan, it doesn't mean you should rush to change your little one's 'schedule' – we use the word 'schedule' very lightly here.

If however, the napping 'schedule' is consistently being fought against by your child then it may be time to drop a nap – it's a sad day when the one and only nap is ready to be given the boot also.

I very clearly recall when my oldest boy was around 2.5 years old, and I had a 2 month old. They napped at the same time for about a month and it was a month of absolute bliss! I could rush around and do a quick tidy then sit down and relax for an hour or so, all by myself! Then my toddler decided he didn't need a nap at all anymore. I'd put him down and he would sing a lovely song of 'I'm awaaaaake' and 'I don't wanna sleeeeeep'. The dual nap dream was over.

Say for example your little one is currently having 3 naps, with 2 hours in between each nap.

As the months go on, this 2 hour gap between naps may start to increase to 2.5 hours.

What this means is that by the time the third nap has taken place, bedtime is pushed out to quite late and you may find your nice quiet peaceful evenings are starting to be encroached on.

You can also get in to a cycle where the late nap and therefore late bedtime leads to not enough sleep at night then the child *needs* the nap to get through the afternoon/evening (generally a later bedtime doesn't lead to a later wake up, it just means less hours sleep at night).

So to drop from three to two naps, or from two to one nap, the best thing to do slowly stretch out the time gap between the naps, and then make bedtime slightly earlier.

Here is an example (these are approximate timings, every baby is different, and every day can be different too!):

Moving from two naps to one nap:

Morning wake: 7am
First Nap: 10.30am
Second Nap: 3pm
Bedtime: 8.30pm

When it is time to drop down to one nap you will find that the first nap becomes a bit of a battle and even though you are putting your little one down at around 10.30am (as per the example above) they are taking a long time to fall asleep.

Try moving this out by half an hour to 11am, this may then push the second nap out by half an hour to 3.30pm and bedtime may even be pushed to 9pm.

After **TWO** days of this, push the morning nap out by another half hour to 11.30am. Then skip the second nap altogether and put your little one to bed at 6.30-7pm.

When the time comes that your little one is getting ready to **drop naps altogether** – around anywhere from around two to three years old (this is an approximate age range only, don't think that just because your little ones friends are dropping naps your child should be ready also) If you feel like your little one still needs a nap, try moving the start time of the nap out by an hour, and wake them up after no more than an hour of sleep, keeping in mind that you don't want their bedtime to be pushed out too late.

There is often a **transition period** where little ones aren't ready to drop the nap altogether, but they don't need the nap every day either. During this time, when the nap battle begins, try to give them the extra nap every second day, and then move to every few days. I find that an additional nap on a Wednesday and a Saturday seems to work well during the **transition period.**

CHAPTER 5 – TRANSITIONING FROM A CRIB TO A BED

Often parents seem in a hurry to move their toddlers from a crib in to a bed. I think it is best to keep them in their crib for a longer period, to around 2.5 - 3 years of age.

The reason for this is that their crib is their safe place, they have spent so much time in there over the past few years, and no matter what else has changed in their world (a lot has been changing!) their crib has been unchanged for the most part.

I advise to leave them in here for as long as possible.

If you have a new baby on the way and want to use the crib for the new baby, then it is even worth buying a second crib rather than moving the older toddler in to the bed too soon. If money does not allow this, then try to make sure you move the toddler in to the bed a good few months before the new baby arrives so that it doesn't seem like the new baby is 'taking' the toddlers crib.

Safety can be an issue. If you have a little Houdini who has figured out they can climb out then this can pose a risk of injury if they fall while climbing out, others can climb out safely. If this is happening then it is time to make the move to the bed.

If you have a crib with a side that can be removed then it can be a good test to see if your toddler is ready to move in to a bed by taking off the side and placing something soft on the ground beneath in case they do roll out.

If they go a few nights of staying in the crib without falling out of the side then they are ready to make the big move!

It can also be a sad time for parents as moving to a bed can feel like their little one is no longer a baby and is growing up, so make sure that you are emotionally ready for the big move also – remember, little ones pick up on your anxiety so be confident.

> *Roll up a towel, or take a foam roller and place down the side of the bed under the bottom sheet to prevent your little one from rolling out of bed*

Keep your routine exactly the same as if they were sleeping in their crib. Remember it's probably more of a big deal for you as the parent that they are moving than for them.

Offer your toddler a quick explanation of the change in sleeping arrangements and leave it at that - I find that if you make a big fuss of it then they expect things to be different and to change. We want to keep bedtime as stable as possible and to keep them feeling safe and secure at night time, as they are used to.

It is a great idea to position in the new bed in the same place in the room as the crib was, this way your toddler won't be disoriented in their room, and you are keeping things as familiar as possible for them.

If they are using a toddler pillow, or always sleep with soft toys or a 'blankie' or some sort, be sure to move these in to the bed too, you want to make the surroundings as similar to their crib as possible.

When it comes to bed time, I suggest picking up your little one if possible and placing them in the bed, as you would pick them up and placing them in their crib. The reason for this is that if you put them in there they should also expect you to take them out, and they may not even realise they can get out by themselves (to start with anyway).

If they are not getting out of the bed but are crying out, then go through **The Five Minute Sleep Method Refresher.** This will get your toddler back on track with falling asleep fairly quickly.

If your little one is getting out of bed – this is a novelty and a new game for some toddlers – then this can cause some issues and create a drawn out bedtime.

Keep a hallway light on just in case they do wake up in the night and wander.

Use **The Staircase Method** if your toddler starts getting out of bed.

The first time they get up, tell them that it is bed time, place them back in to bed, say good night and leave.

Each time they get up after this, simply pick them up without saying anything, place them back in to bed, give them a reassuring kiss and leave.

You may be up and down and up and down with them many many times for the first couple of nights, but sticking to this method, and not making a fuss of them when they get out of bed and come out will let them know fairly quickly that there is no point in getting up. They won't get the attention they are wanting.

This transition doesn't have to be stressful, and as mentioned it is probably more of a big deal to you as the parent than for your little one.

CHAPTER 6 – MANAGING DAYLIGHT SAVINGS

Just when you have the sleep timings sorted, and napping and bedtime is going well, Day Light Savings rolls around and mucks it all up again!

There is also a relatively easy fix for this though so don't panic!

You can either start preparing for this a few days out so that the timings are right or just wait until the changeover date.

Daylight Savings Starting
When Daylight Savings starts the clocks go forwards one hour during Spring.
This means that if your little one is going to bed at 7pm, when the new time changes over 7pm will be 6pm in the old time. It is likely they will resist going to bed an hour earlier, and will wake up early in the morning if their body clocks haven't had time to adjust.

Whenever you decide to start, using my **Five Day Daylight Savings Method** is an easy way to have your little one adjust:

Day 1 : Put your little one down for their last nap 15 minutes earlier and wake them up 15 minutes earlier, then put them to bed 15 minutes earlier than usual.

Day 2 : Put your little one down for their last nap 15 minutes earlier and wake them up 15 minutes earlier, then put them to bed 15 minutes earlier than usual.

Day 3 : Put your little one down for their last nap 30 minutes earlier and wake them up 30 minutes earlier, then put them to bed 30 minutes earlier than usual.

Day 4 : Put your little one down for their last nap 45 minutes earlier and wake them up 45 minutes earlier, then put them to bed 45 minutes earlier than usual.

Day 5 : Put your little one down for their last nap 60 minutes earlier and wake them up 60 minutes earlier, then put them to bed 60 minutes earlier than usual.

It can be harder getting children to sleep when it is still light outside, so investing in some blackout curtains or blinds is very useful also.

Daylight Savings Ending
When Daylight Savings ends the clocks go backwards one hour during Fall.

This means that if your little one is going to bed at 7pm, when the new time changes over 7pm will be 8pm in the old time so it is likely they will be over tired going to bed an hour later. They will also be tired in the morning as their body clocks haven't had time to adjust

Whenver you decide to start, using my **Five Day Daylight Savings Method** is an easy way to have your little one adjust:

Day 1 : Put your little one down for their last nap 15 minutes earlier and wake them up 15 minutes earlier, then put them to bed 15 minutes earlier than usual.

Day 2 : Put your little one down for their last nap 15 minutes earlier and wake them up 15 minutes earlier, then put them to bed 15 minutes earlier than usual.

Day 3 : Put your little one down for their last nap 30 minutes earlier and wake them up 30 minutes earlier, then put them to bed 30 minutes earlier than usual.

Day 4 : Put your little one down for their last nap 45 minutes earlier and wake them up 45 minutes earlier, then put them to bed 45 minutes earlier than usual.

Day 5 : Put your little one down for their last nap 60 minutes earlier and wake them up 60 minutes earlier, then put them to bed 60 minutes earlier than usual.

CHAPTER 7 – CONCLUSION

Being a parent is often hard.

There *may* be nights where you are up and down and up and down with your little ones, and this *will* go on for a few years **BUT** you are now armed with the tools to make this easier and your little one now knows how to fall asleep quickly and on their own.

For the most part your child should be sleeping soundly and thriving.

Illnesses, growing pains and general life will *sometimes* get in the way of a good night's sleep. This is just part of being a parent.

If you are having a bad day or two try to remember the positive things about your child. And remember how far you have come with the sleepless nights.

Every day write down three positive things that have happened on that day or three things that you are grateful for. Keep this list ongoing so that you can look back over it and realise that your child is precious and that life is great!

Remember to get out and get some fresh air as much as possible, keep fit and look after yourself so that you can be the best parent you can be this is the greatest gift you can give your children.

Communicate with your partner, talk about your strategies as parents and what you want for your children.

Make friends with other parents and share ideas, don't judge others on their parenting techniques. Just as children are unique, there are many different ways to raise children so try to be supportive.

ENJOY this time with them as children. Get down and play with them, playing is learning. The tidying can wait another day, go to the park, bake, get crafty, get messy. If the housework is getting you down then try to make a fun game out of it and get them to help.

And lastly, be **CONSISTANT** and **CONFIDENT** in your ability as a parent. You know what is best for your little one.

'Children Learn What They Live'

If a child lives with criticism, he learns to condemn.

If a child lives with hostility, he learns to fight. If a child lives with ridicule, he learns to be shy.

If a child learns to feel shame, he learns to feel guilty. If a child lives with tolerance, he learns to be patient.

If a child lives with encouragement he learns confidence.

If a child lives with praise, he learns to appreciate.

If a child lives with fairness, he learns justice.

If a child lives with security, he learns to have faith. If a child lives with approval, he learns to like himself.

If a child lives with acceptance and friendship, he learns to find love in the world.

EXTRA – PARENTING TIPS, TRICKS & QUOTES

- "Always kiss your kids goodnight, even if they're already asleep" - H. Jackson Brown, Jr

- Save time and money on nappies by checking the wet indicator on the front of the nappy before changing (most quality nappies will have this indicator).

- Use the 'envelope folds' on baby clothes to easily pull tops *down* to take off when they have spilled or pooed, this avoids spreading the mess.

- "Don't worry that children never listen to you, worry that they are always watching you" – Robert Fulghum

- Massaging a baby is a great way to calm and sooth before bedtime.

- Give your little ones as much fresh air as possible every day.

- When bathing newborns, swaddle them in a light cotton wrap to help them feel secure before lowering them in to the water and slowing unwrapping them.

- "Your children will become what you are, so be what you want them to be" – David Bly

- Add a few drops of lavender oil to the bath water to relax your little one before bedtime.

- To help relieve gas in baby's tummy, hold their feet and gently move their knees up to their chest and down again. Using a cycling motion works well too.

- "Your children need your presence more than your presents" - Jesse Jackson

- If you're taking toddlers or children to a crowded venue or event, make a bracelet with your phone number on it, or simply write your number on their arm in case they become lost or separated.

- Before going shoe shopping for children, draw the outline of their foot on a piece of paper and take it with you – this way you'll always get a shoe that fits whether your little one is not willing to try on the shoes or if they aren't with you.

- "A baby will make love stronger, days shorter, nights longer, bankroll smaller, home happier, clothes shabbier, the past forgotten and the future worth living" – Anonymous

- Giving medicine to little ones can be hard work and even a little traumatic. Cut the tip off an old pacifier and put liquid medicine in here to administer it, then they can simply suck on the pacifier and receive the required dose.

- Put a cupcake patty or takeaway coffee lid on the stick under a popsicle to stop the drips and avoid a big mess.

- "You don't always know what your kids will do, but your kids should always know what you will do" – Joyce Sanders

- When talking to children try to talk using positive words rather than negative, for example, avoid saying 'Don't do stand up in the bath' instead saying 'Let's sit down in the bath to stay safe'.

- After cutting an apple or orange, hold it back together with a rubberband to take out and eat on the go without it going brown or dry.

- Try to focus on what your kids are doing well - make a fuss when they do something good or right rather than making a big deal and giving too much attention to what they have done wrong or when they misbehave.

- Use your children's paintings as gift wrap for presents for friends and family.

- Enjoy your children, time is precious.

65994236R00064

Made in the USA
Lexington, KY
31 July 2017